MW01620676

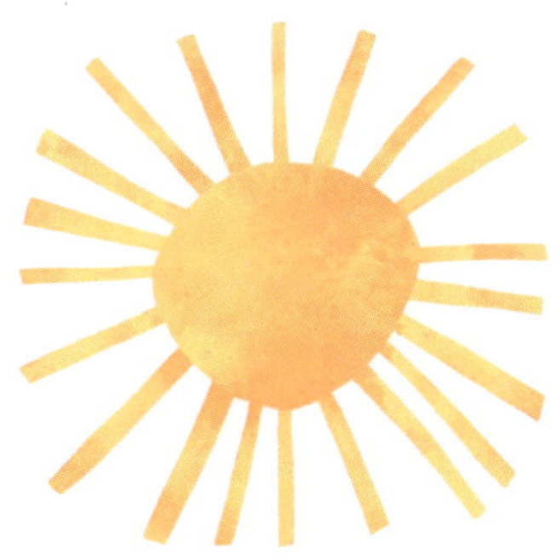

Praise for
Tell Me About...

"This is an important birth narrative for every adopted child to have and to hold. It is a keepsake from their first mother, their birthmother. It is affirmimg for an adoptee to know she cared enough to write in a journal like this and share knowledge about their "genetic inheritance" as someting to be valued and not shamed. **I highly recommend this book for all birth mothers who have made a consensual decision to place their child for adoption."**

-Jeanette Yoffe
Licensed Marriage and Family Therapist
Founder of Celia Center, Non-Profit Adoption Foster Care Support

"Knowing our origins is integral to building and embracing our identity. The entry-point into life for most adoptees in miracle... and an endless kaleidoscope of unknowns. Imaginings about ourselves that live on far past our childhood and that may never be filled in. Abigail and Laurie have delicately tapped into the heart of the adoptee and with this book have built a bridge for birth-mothers and adoptees to discover themselves in ways so many take for granted. This is the definition of priceless gift. I am so grateful it has arrived. **I wish only that my birth-mother could have that copy."**

-Jonathan Nadlman
Licensed Marriage and Family Therapist

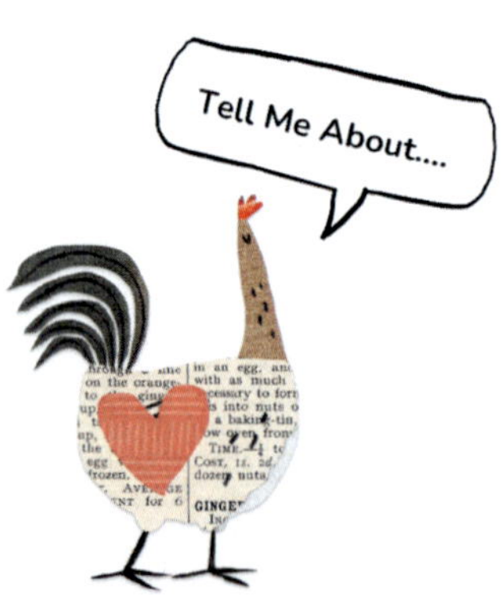
Tell Me About....

TELL ME ABOUT MY
Birth Mother

A journal about beginnings

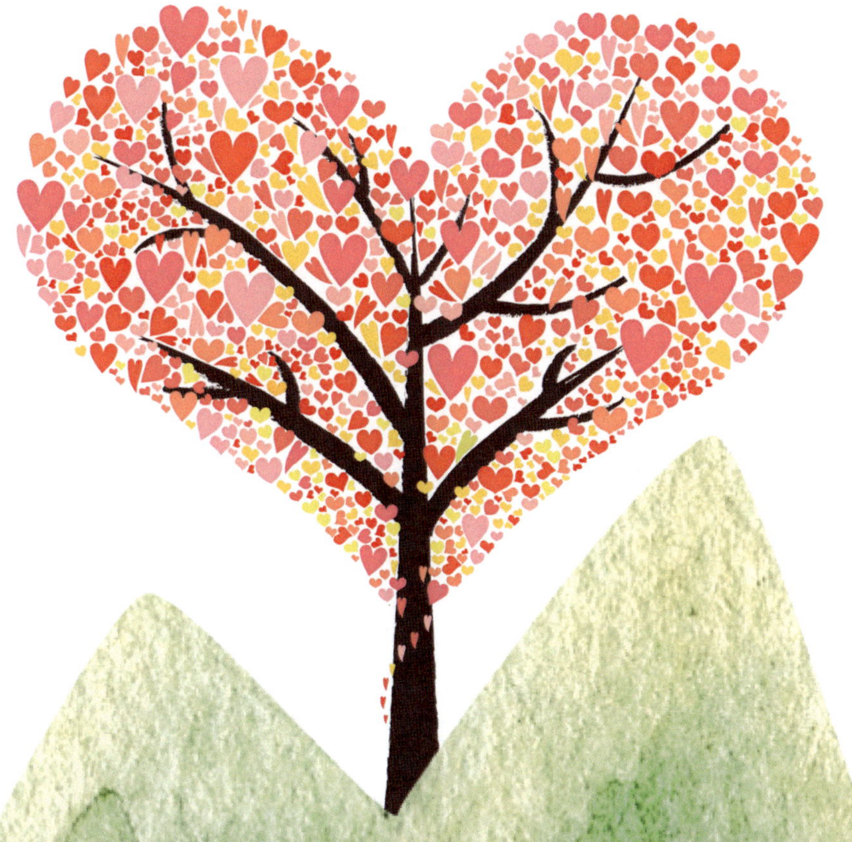

Abigail Glass, LMFT & Laurie Shiers, PCC

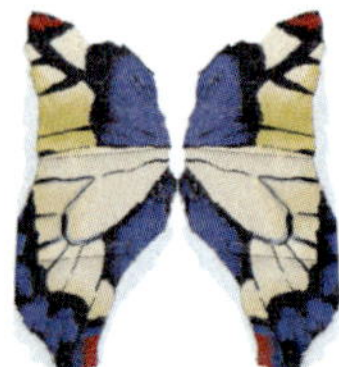

Published by Brainchild Creative in the United States
Cover Design by Laurie Shiers

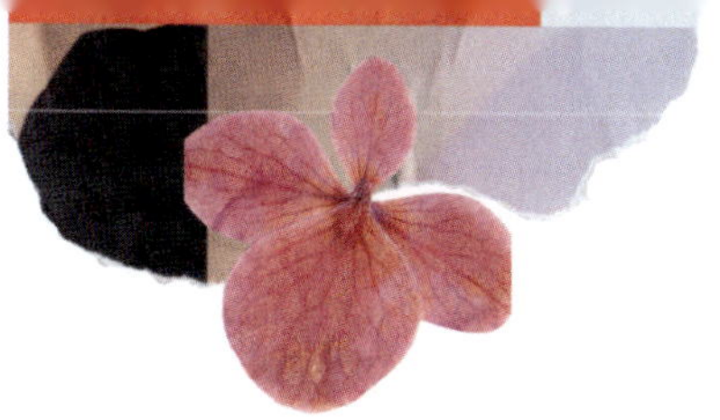

Dear Birth Mother,

We see you and we honor your journey. That's why we created this little book. Our hope is that writing in it will be helpful, and also remind you of some of the wonderful things that make you, well, YOU. This book is designed to be a keepsake for your baby. Filling it in may seem like a small gesture right now, but the details you are about to share will be precious to your child who will read it one day.

When you are ready, please take a deep breath, and go through the pages at your own pace. The questions are open ended enough for you to share as much or as little as you wish. If you don't know an answer, fill in what you DO know. Please remember, however you respond to these questions is just right. Simply be yourself. And if there's something you don't want to answer or doesn't apply to you, feel free to skip the prompt or change it into something you'd rather share.

Thank you, beautiful soul, for sharing your story on these pages. You are a gift, and the book you are holding in your hand right now will also become a treasured gift for your child.

With love and appreciation,
Abby and Laurie

P.S. Need some guidance? Look in the back of this book for ideas on what you might want to include.

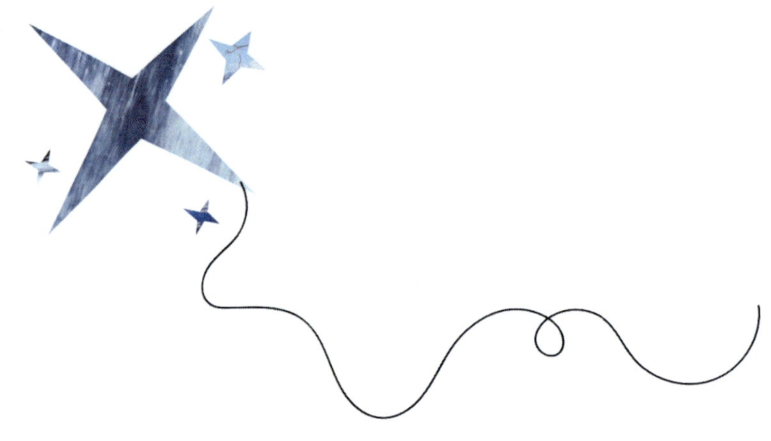

This book is for

____

By

____

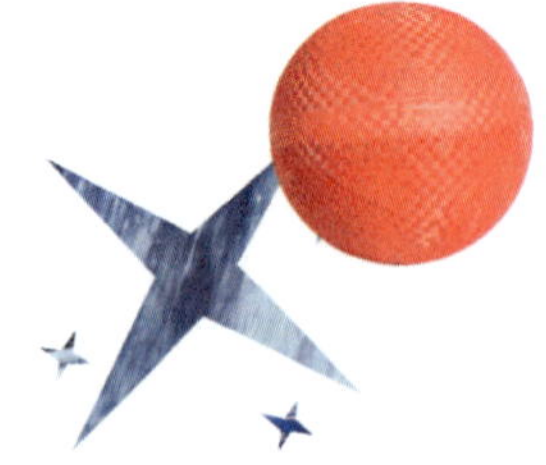

Hello,

BAby

Let me tell you
the beginning of your story

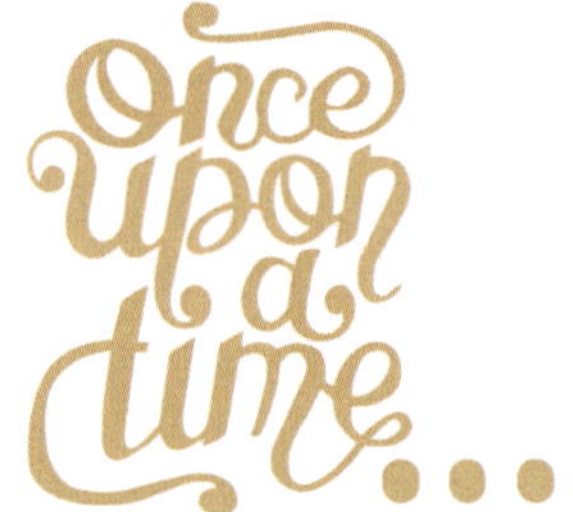

You were born on:

in:

and.......

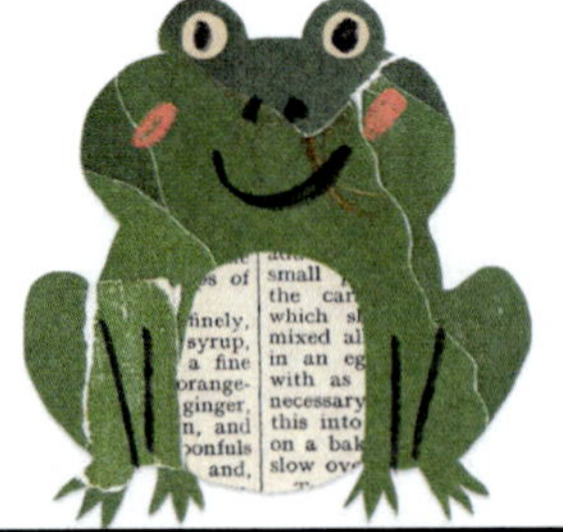

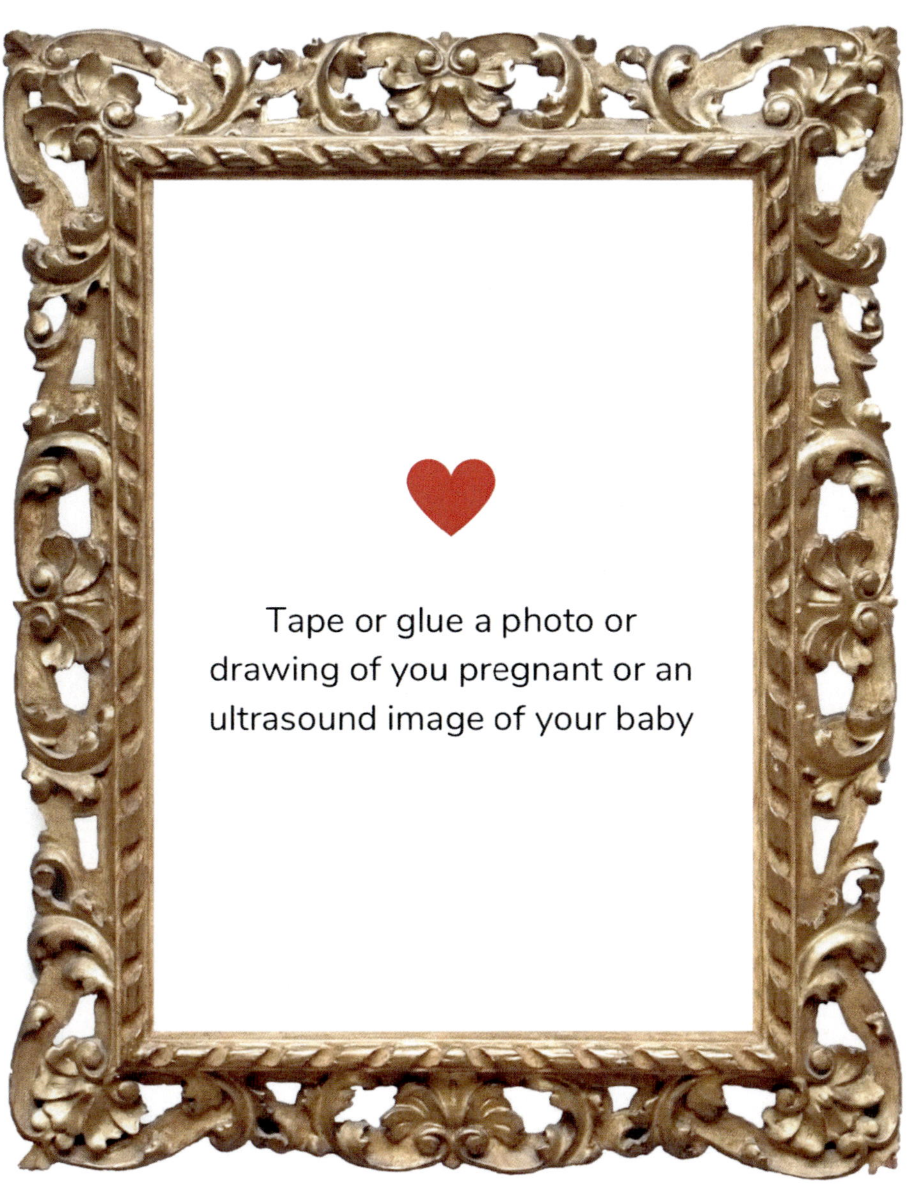

Tape or glue a photo or
drawing of you pregnant or an
ultrasound image of your baby

Here you are!

When you were in my belly,...

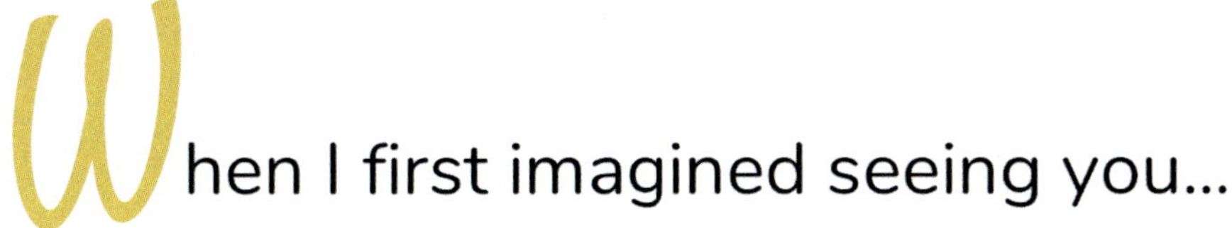

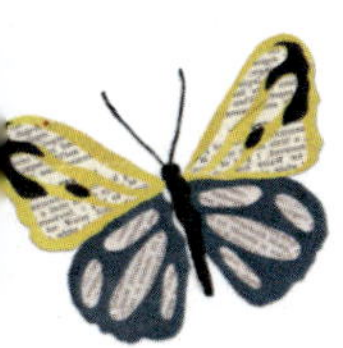

YOU TOOK MY BREATH AWAY

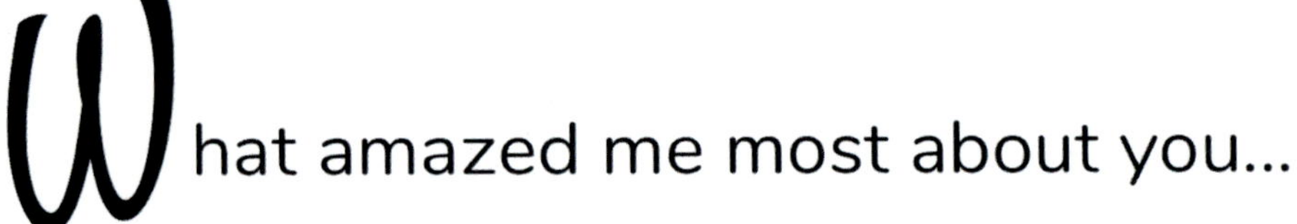

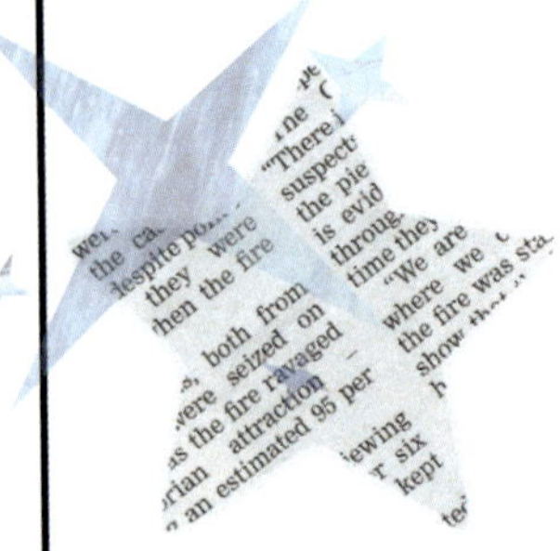

THERE'S ONLY ONE YOU!

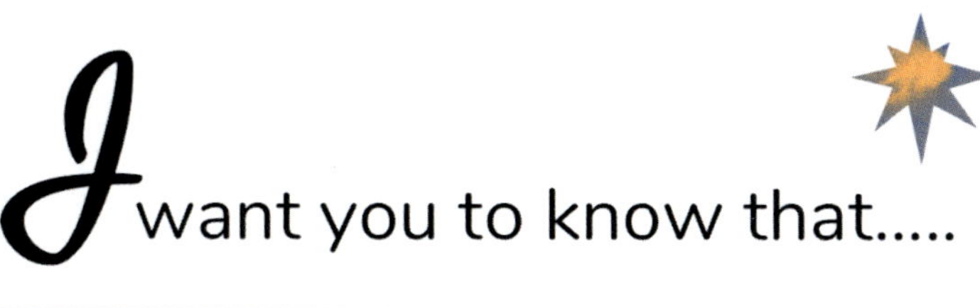
I want you to know that.....

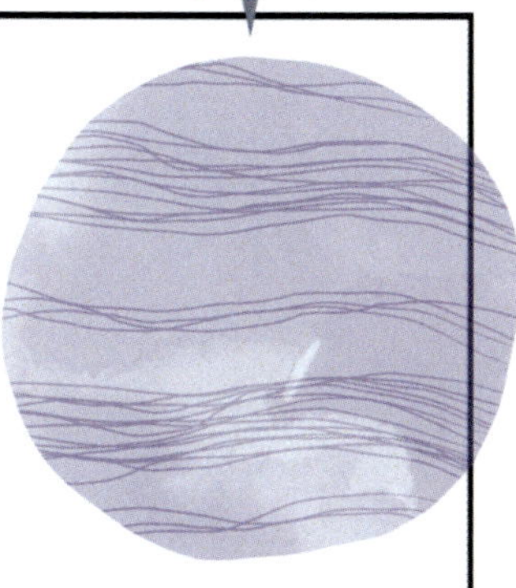

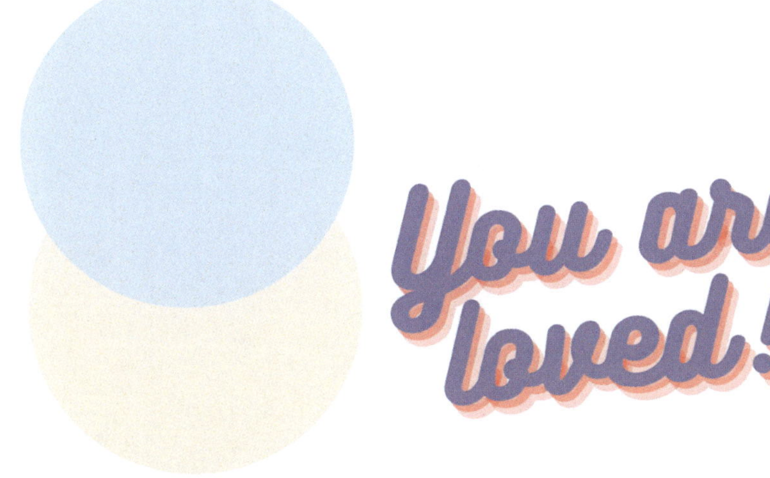
You are loved!

Here's where I lived when
I was pregnant with you....

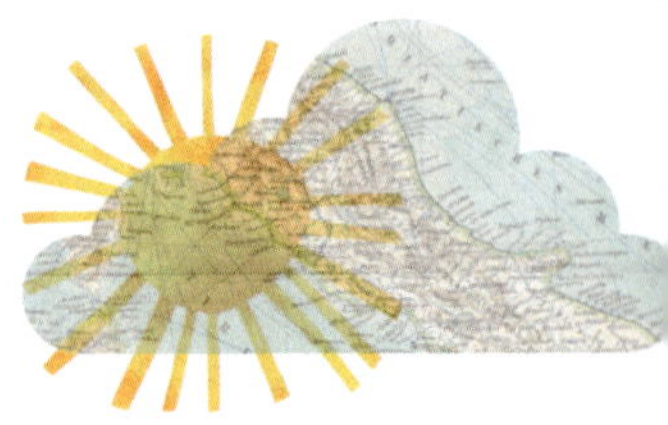

Here are some of the other places we have been....

This is what I know about what's next for you...

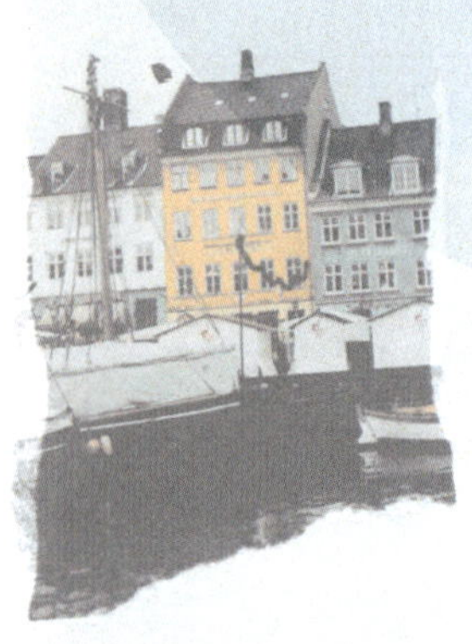

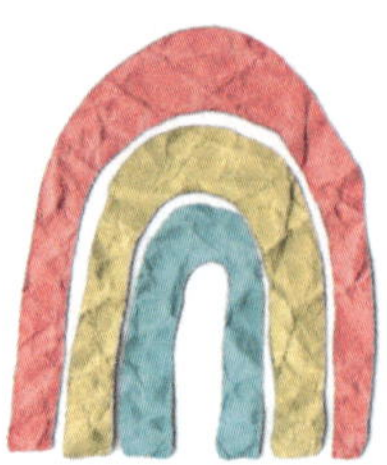

My hopes and dreams for you are.....

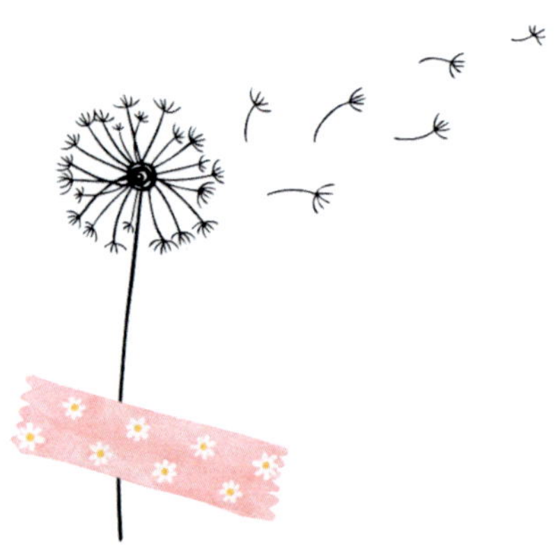

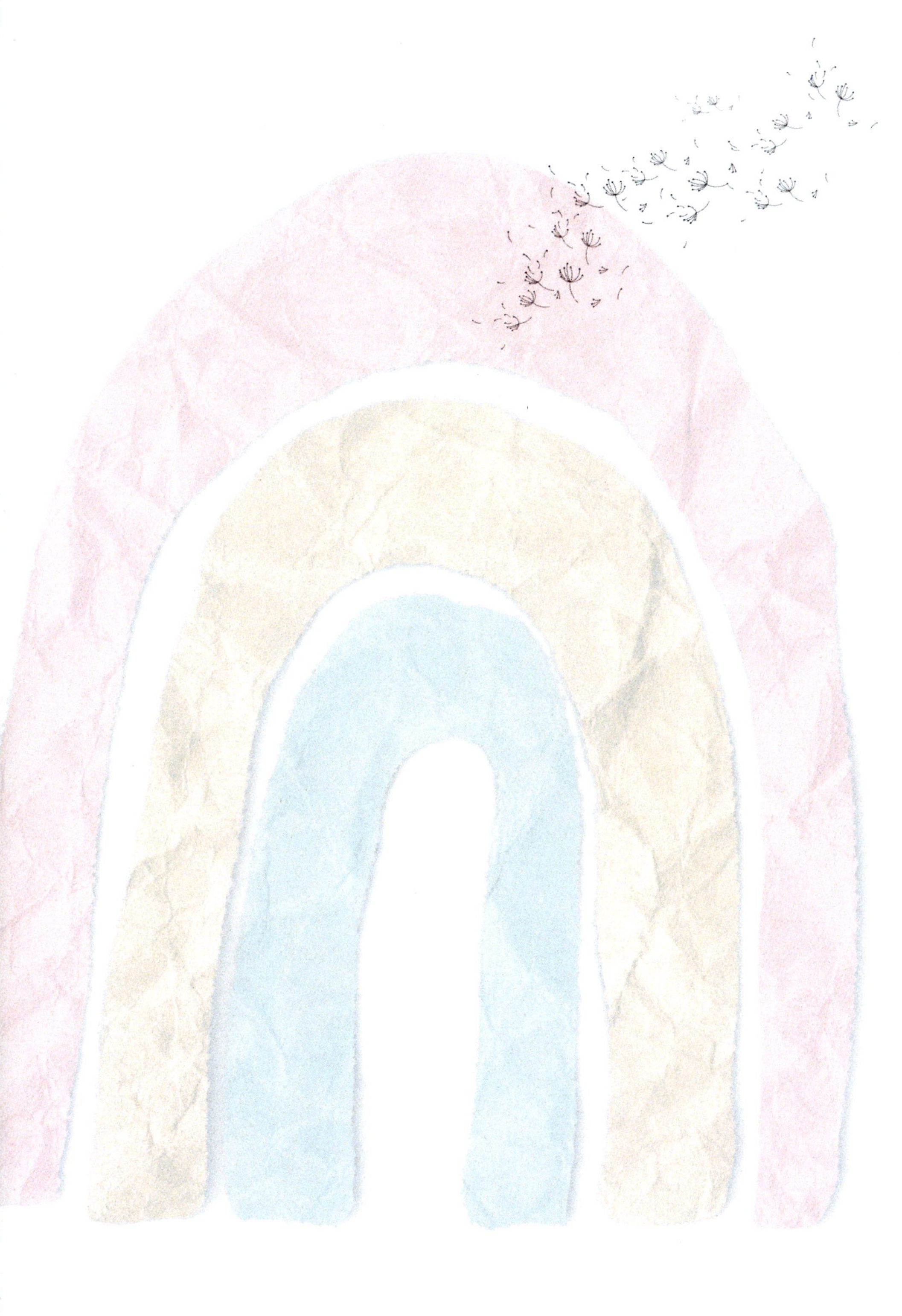

Never forget that....

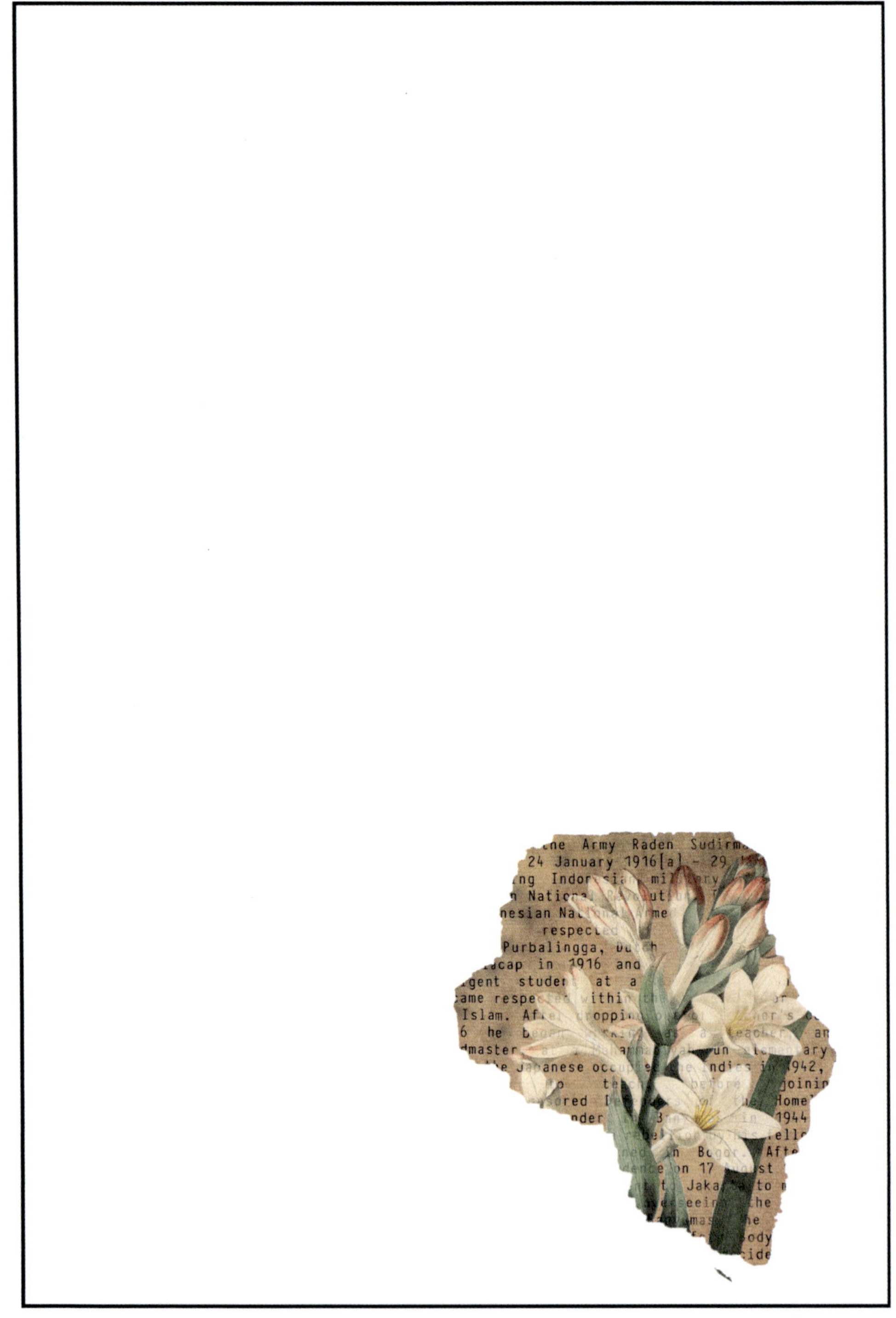

Please always remember....

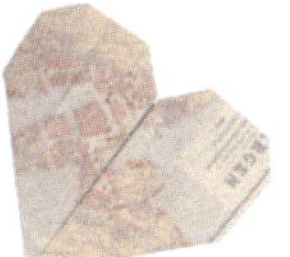

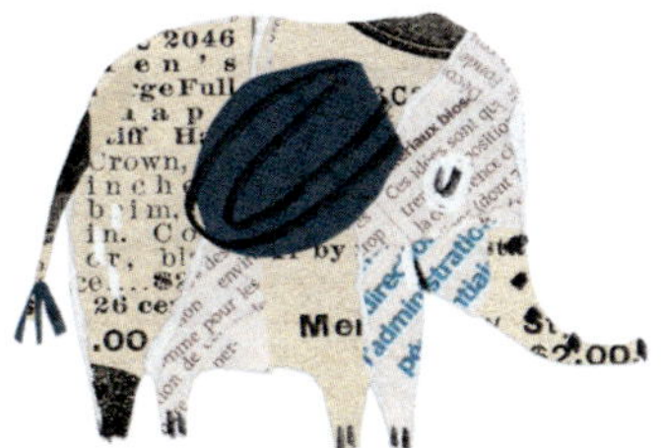

I LOVE YOU.

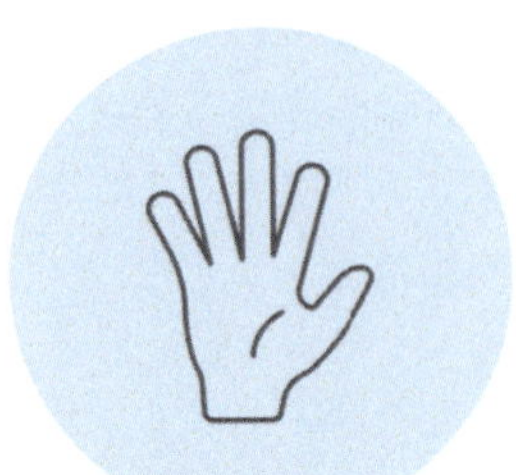

Here's an outline of my hand

Go ahead and trace your hand on this page.

Feel free to color it in!

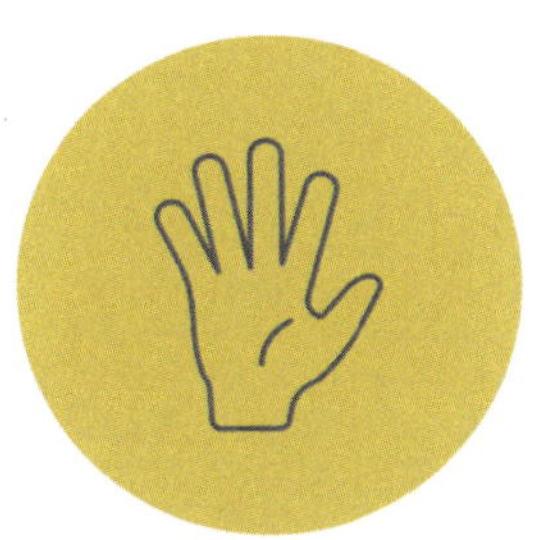

Here's an outline of your hand

Trace your baby's hand or your baby's hand can be traced here later.

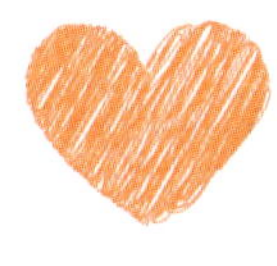

PART TWO

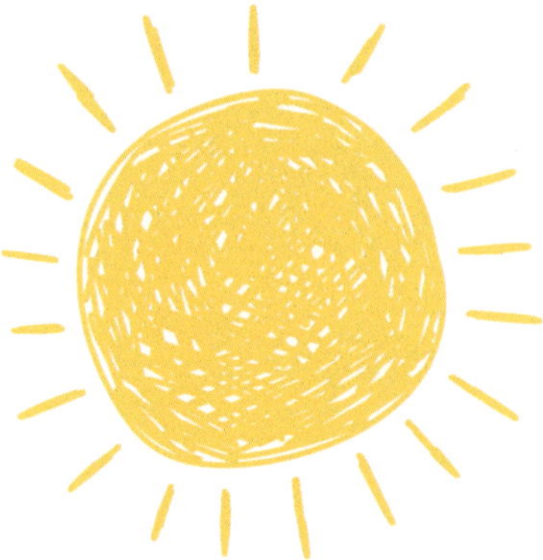

Alright, Kiddo

Now I want to tell you a little bit about me.

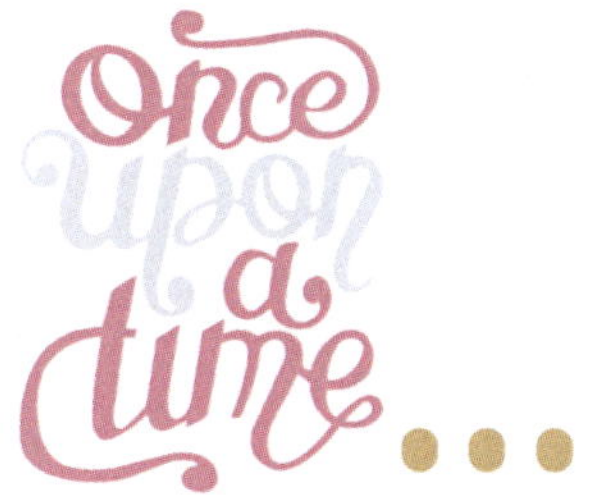

I was born on:

in:

and.......

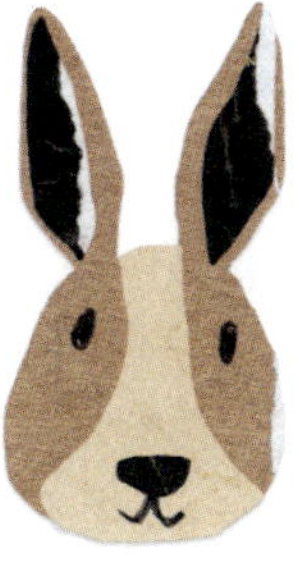

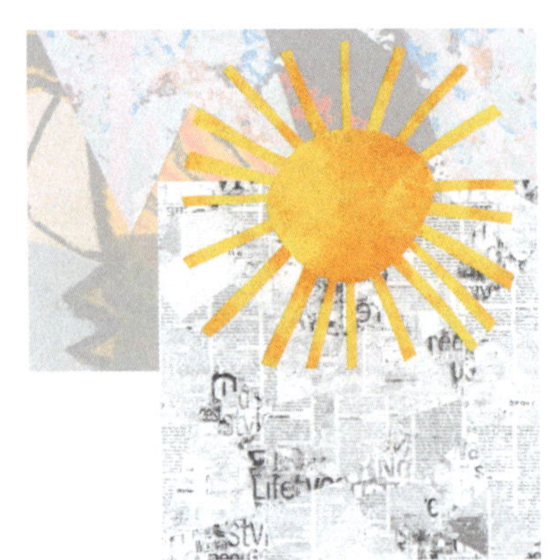

My ethnicity is:

My nationality is:

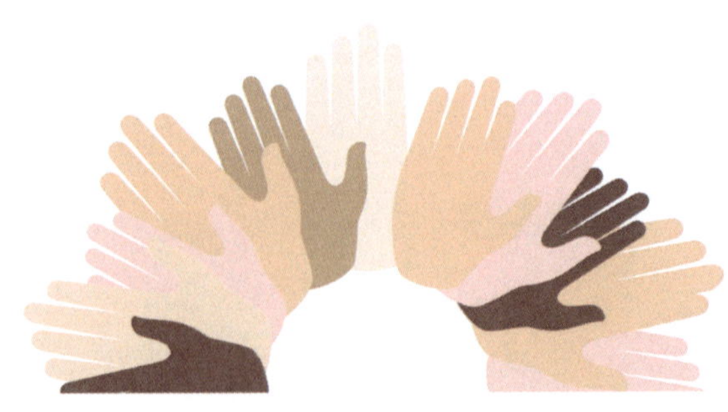

Some of my cultural traditions are.....

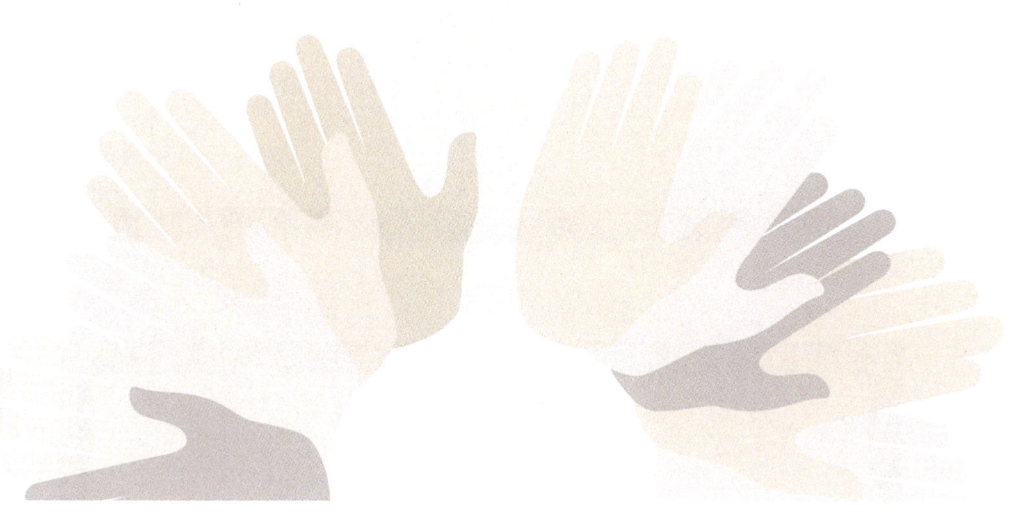

Here I am!

Tape or glue a baby photo or drawing of you here

Then

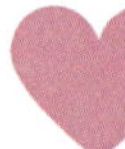

Tape or glue a recent photo or drawing of you here

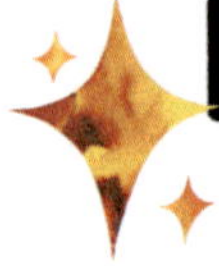

Now

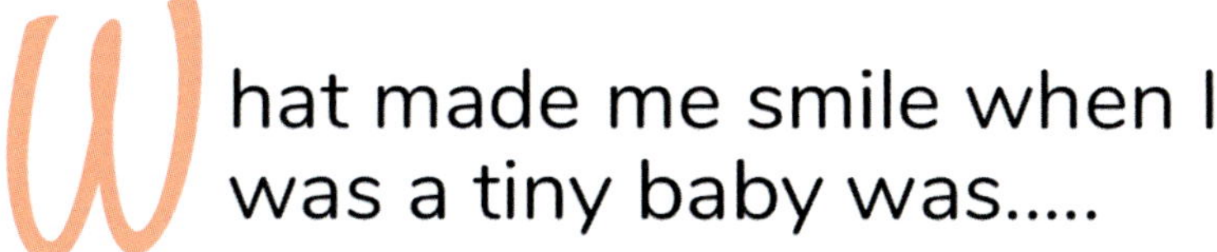

What made me smile when I was a tiny baby was.....

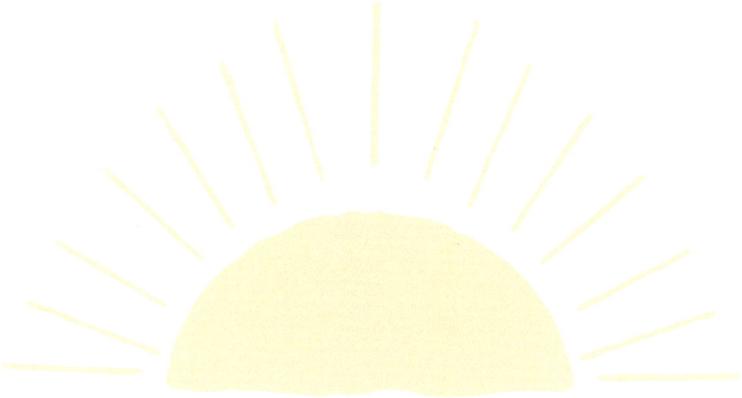

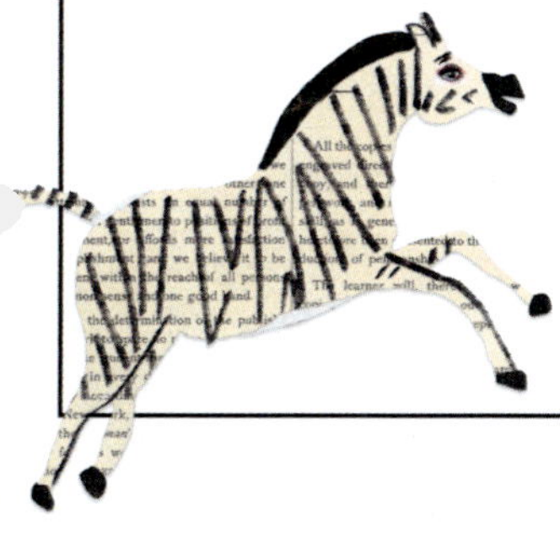

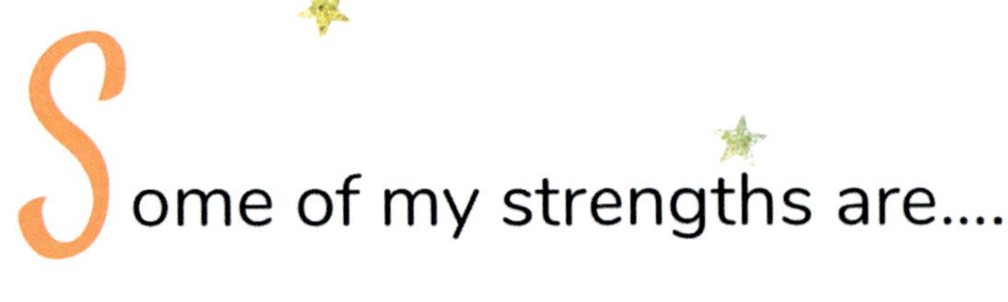

Talents I have.....

Sports I have played....

Here's what I loved to do when I was little:

As a teenager, I....

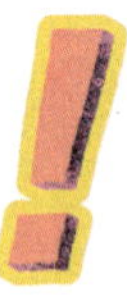

These days, some of my favorite things are...

Some people *describe* me as.....

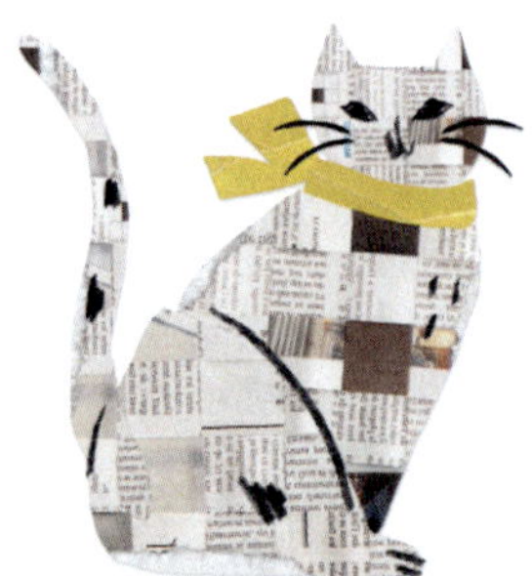

I describe *myself* as....

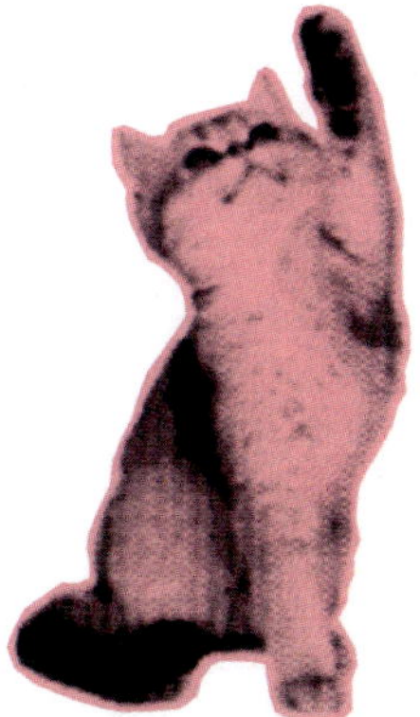

I'm really *Good* at....

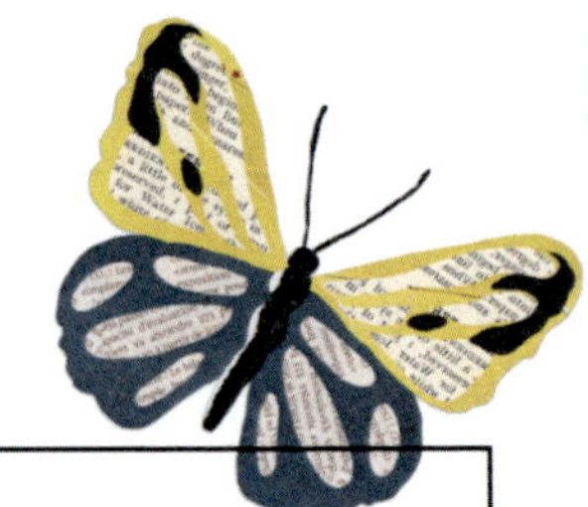

I'm *happiest* when.....

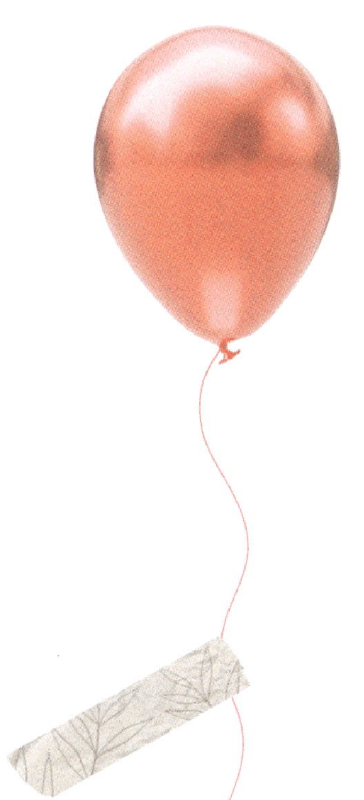

I'm most *proud* of...

To be honest....

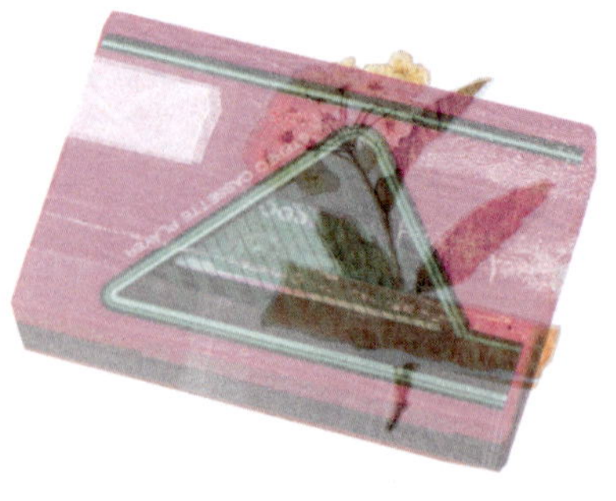

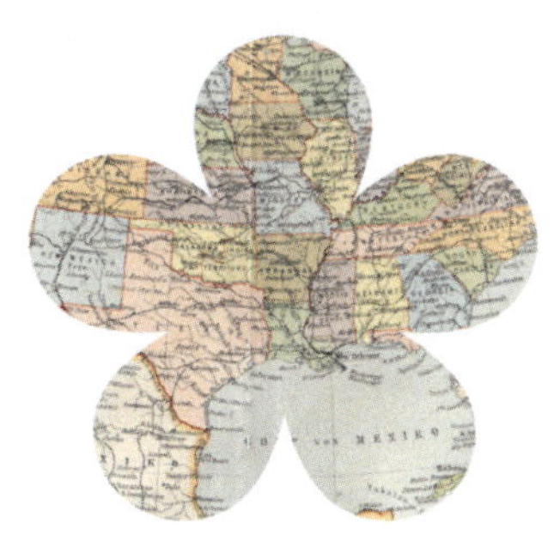

(What you might be surprised to know about me is...)

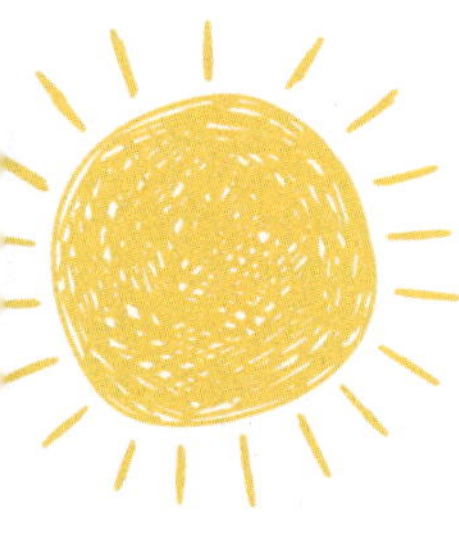

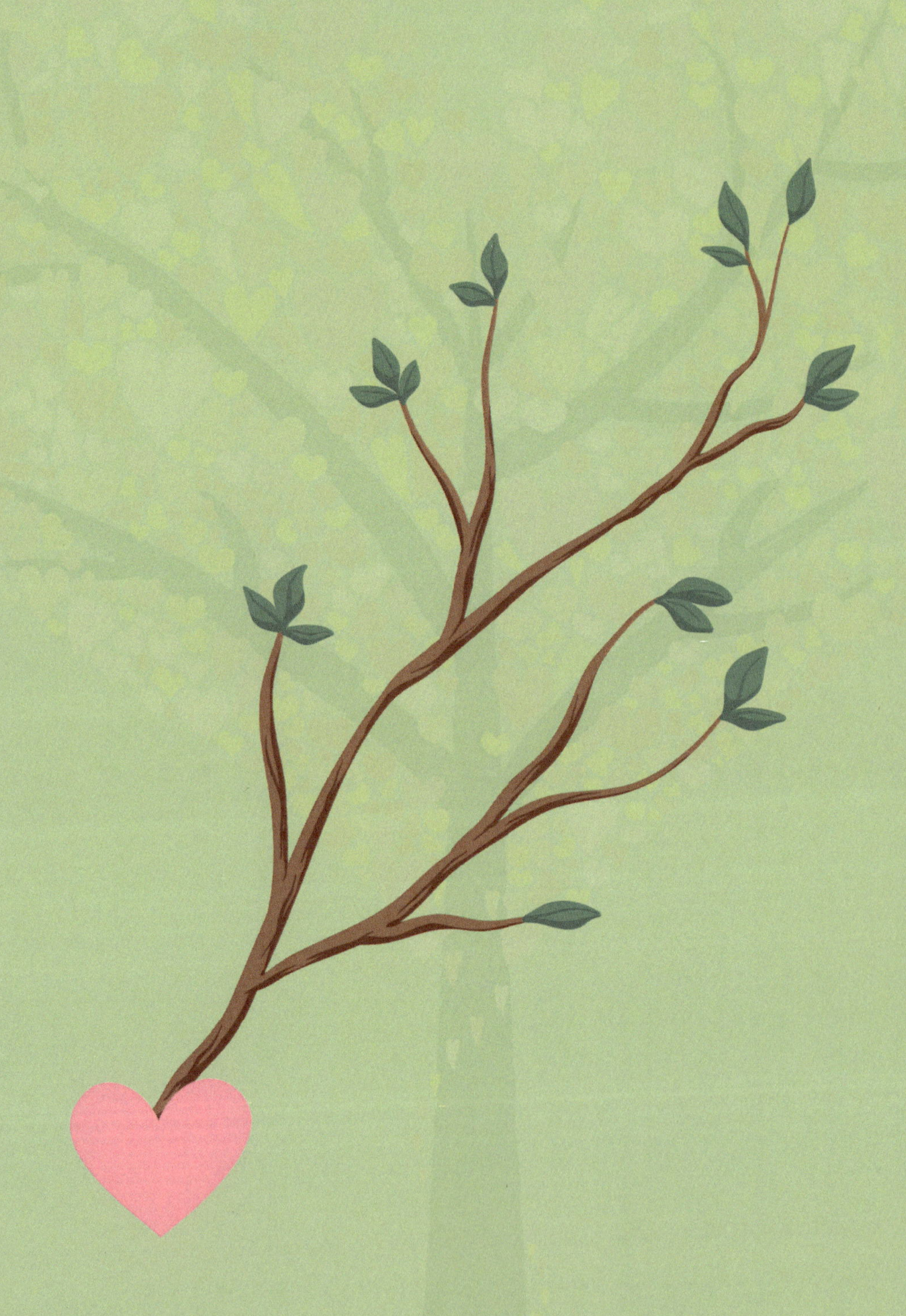

Here are some branches on our Family Tree:

Feel free to add names of other family members including any siblings, aunts, uncles, or cousins around the tree and anywhere on these pages.

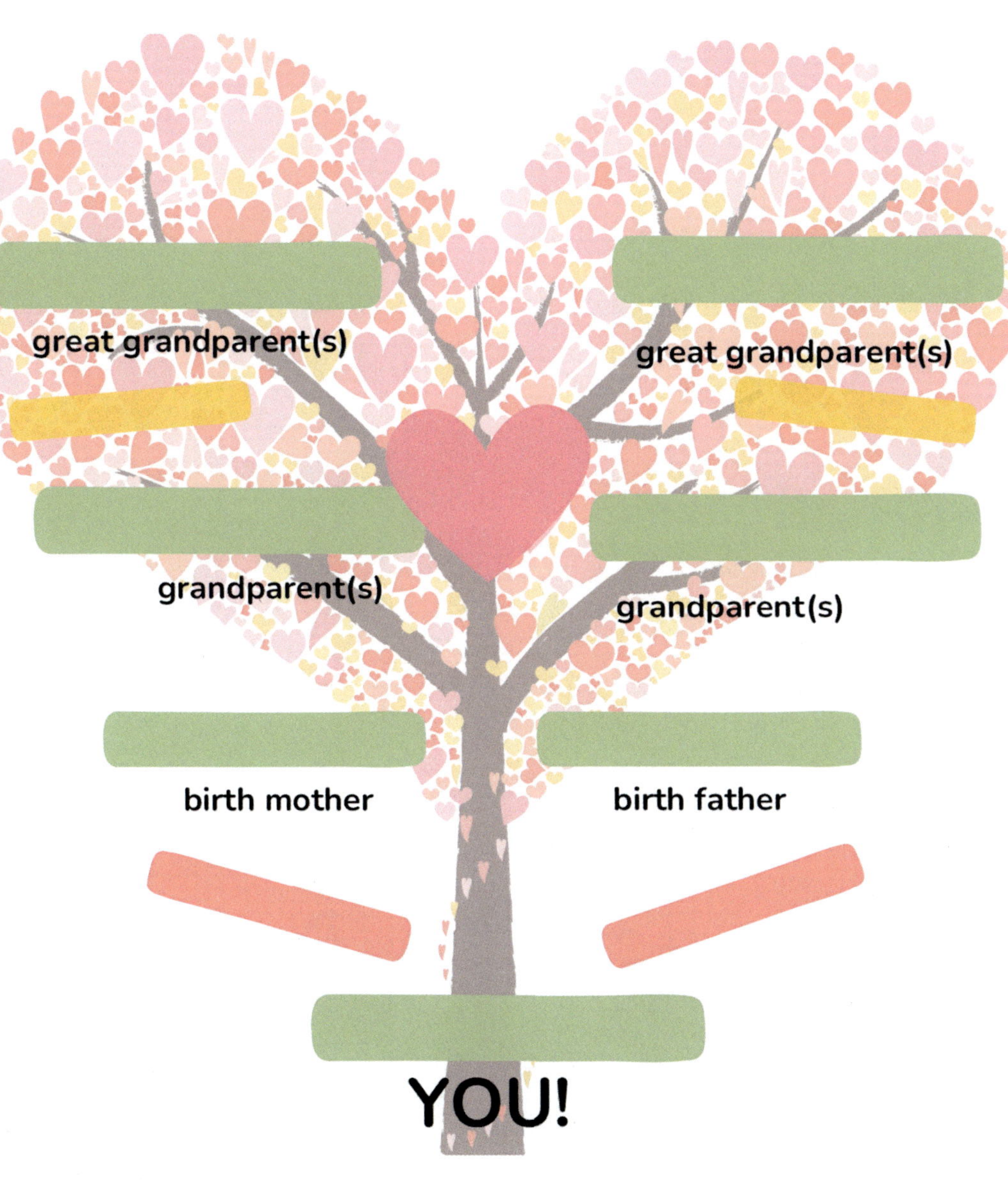

Words of wisdom especially for you:

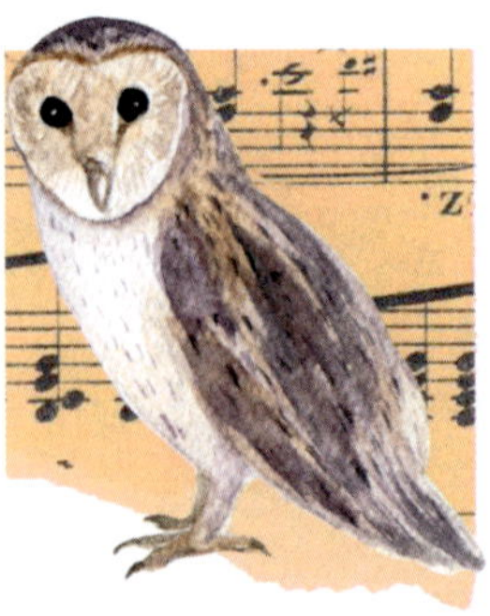

Here is a doodle I made for you:

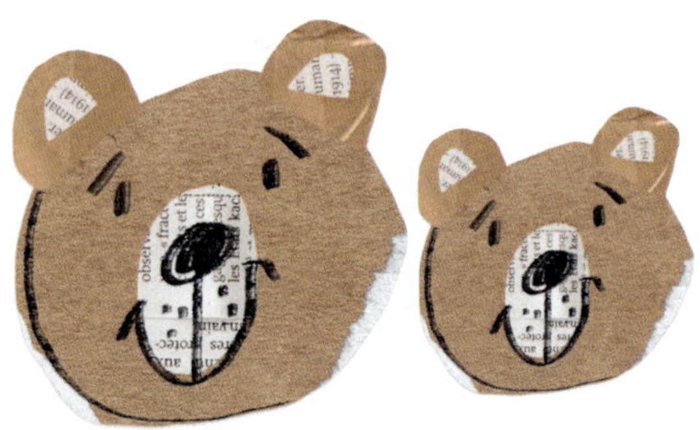

The next pages belong to both of you. Feel free to add whatever you wish: stories, wishes, drawings, photos-- anything you'd like to share about yourself or your journey. When your baby is older, they can add whatever they'd like too!

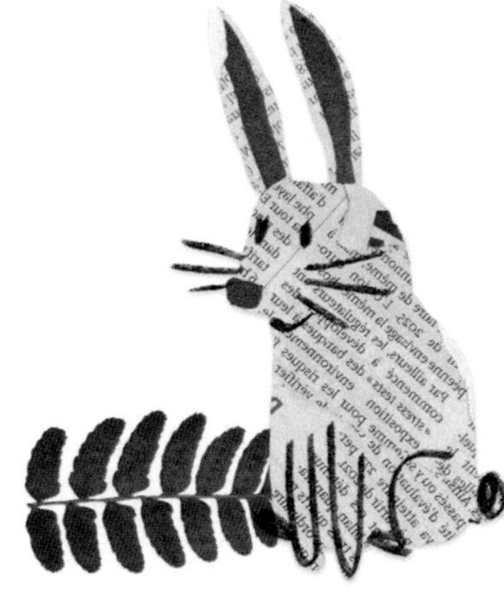

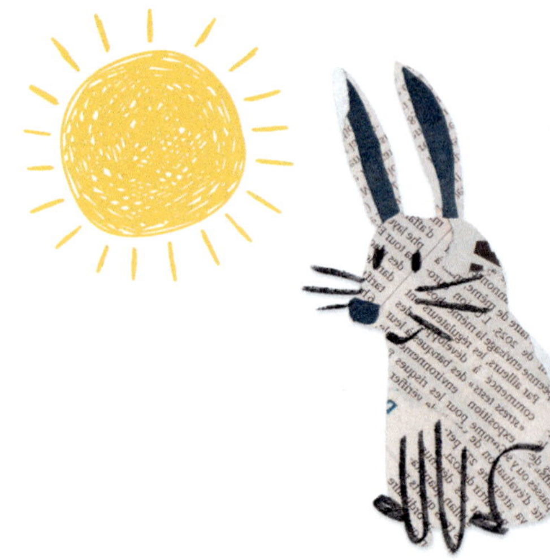

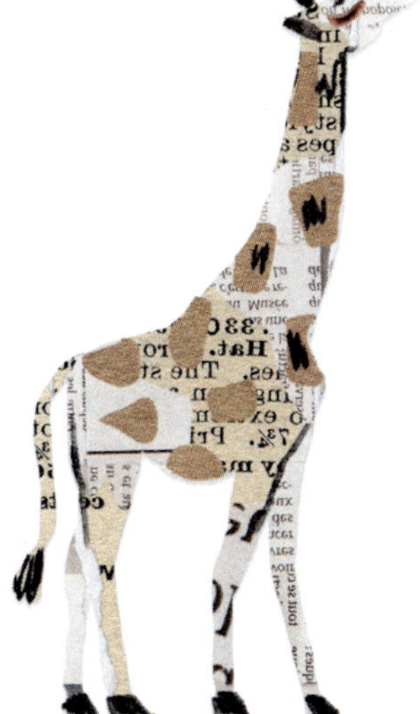

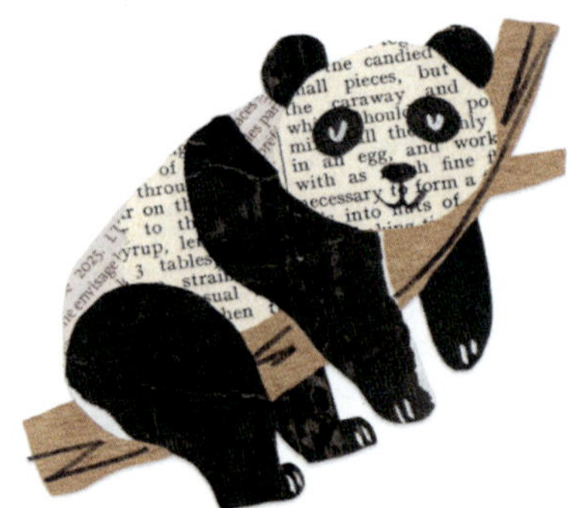

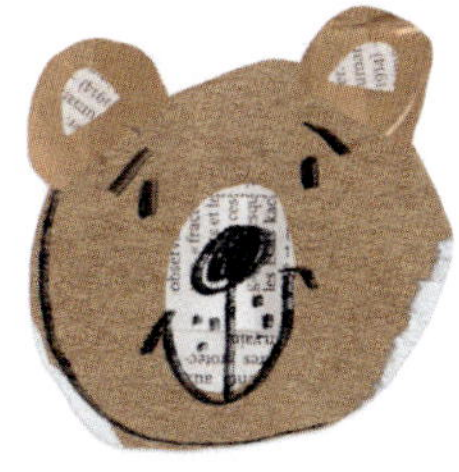

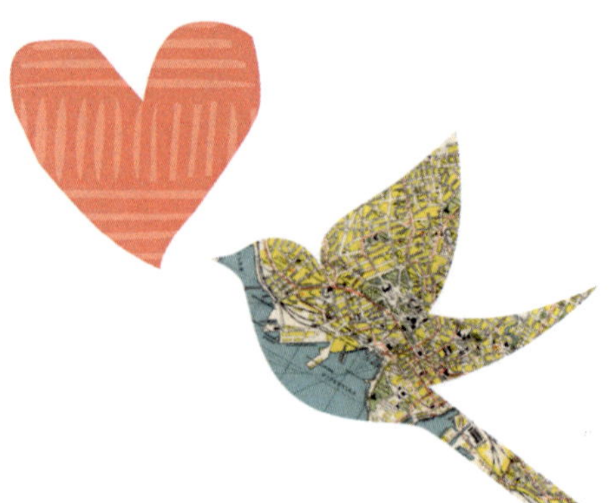

on the orange-
to the ginger
up, lemon,
tables
up, str
the us
egg whe the
frozen.
AVERAGE
for 6
in an egg, an
with as much
necessary to for
is into nuts o
on a baking-tin,
slow oven from
TIME.—¼ to
COST, 1s. 2d.
dozen nuts.
GINGE

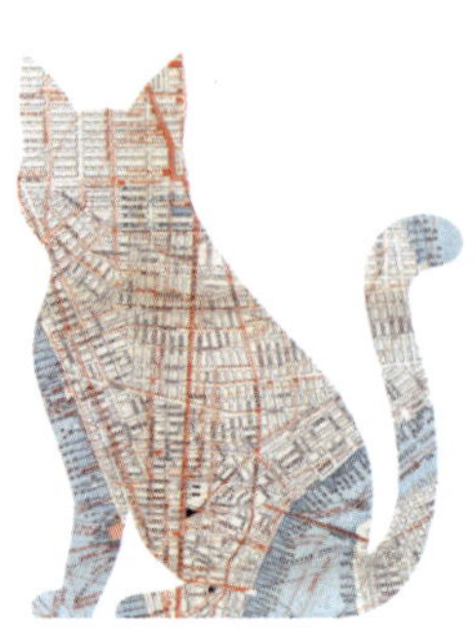

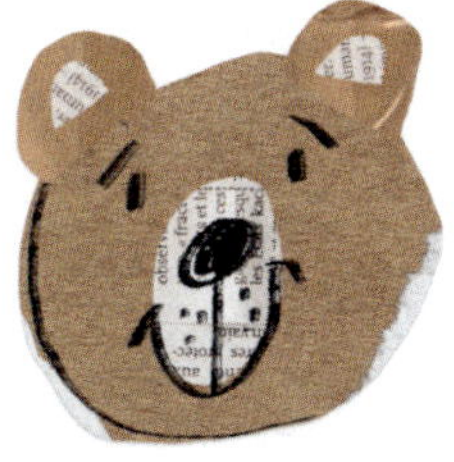

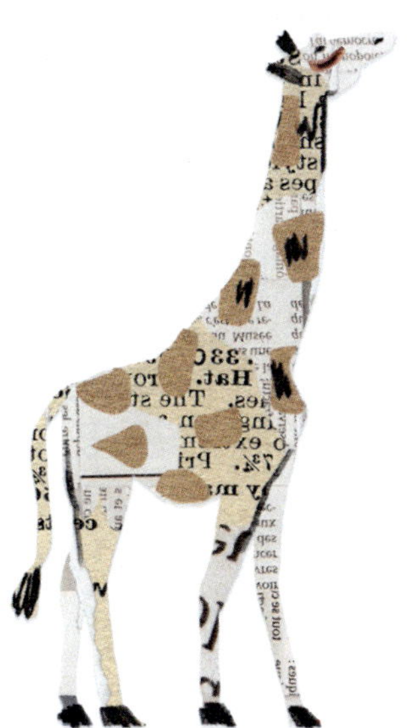

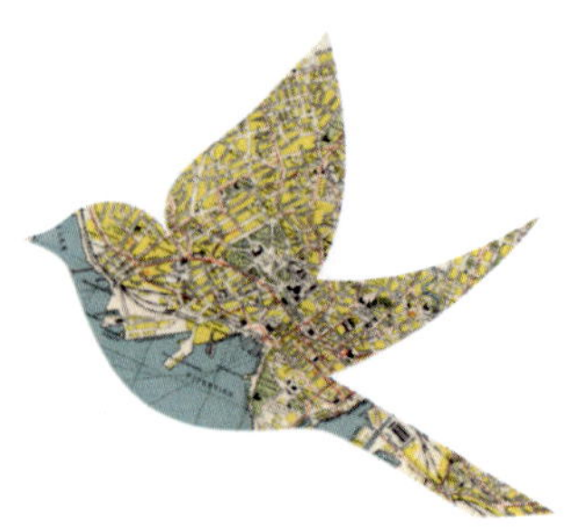

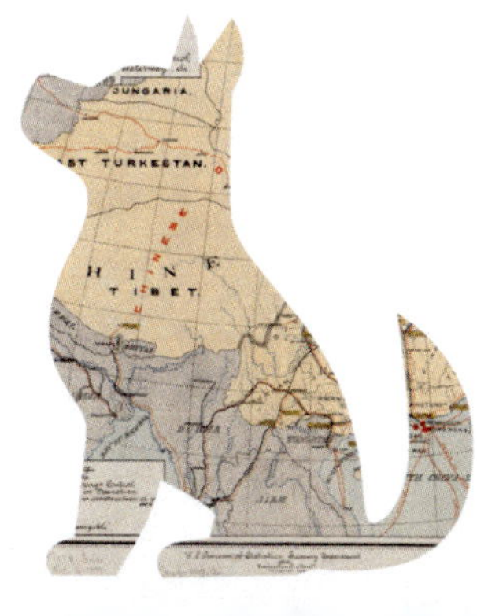
JUNGARIA.
ST TURKESTAN.

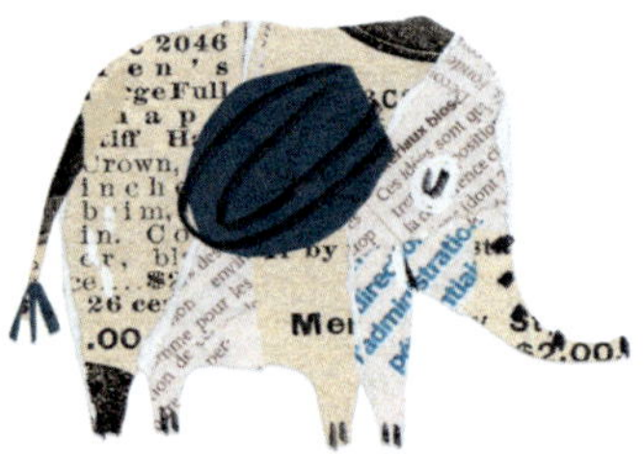

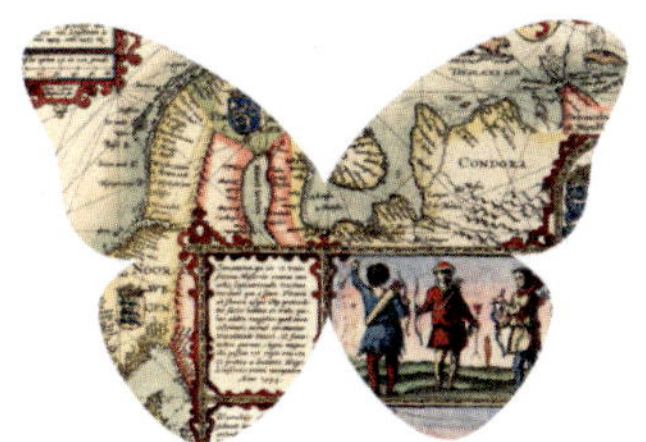
CONDORA

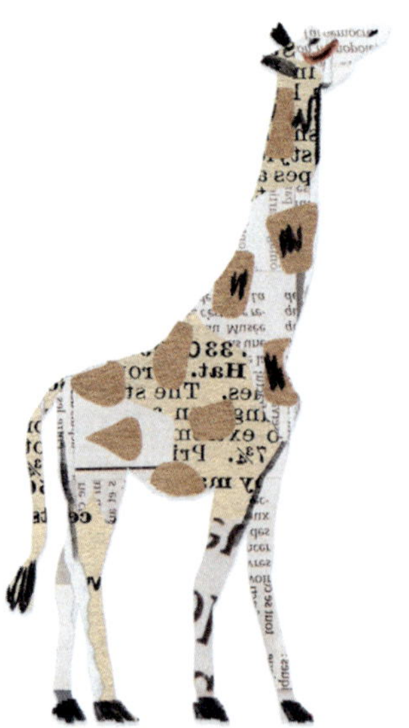

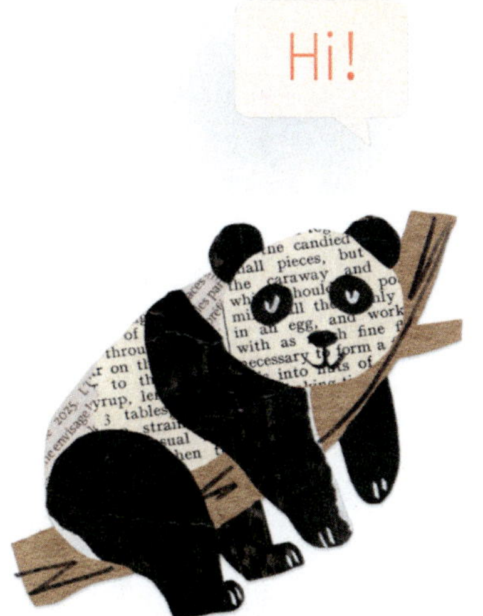
Hi!

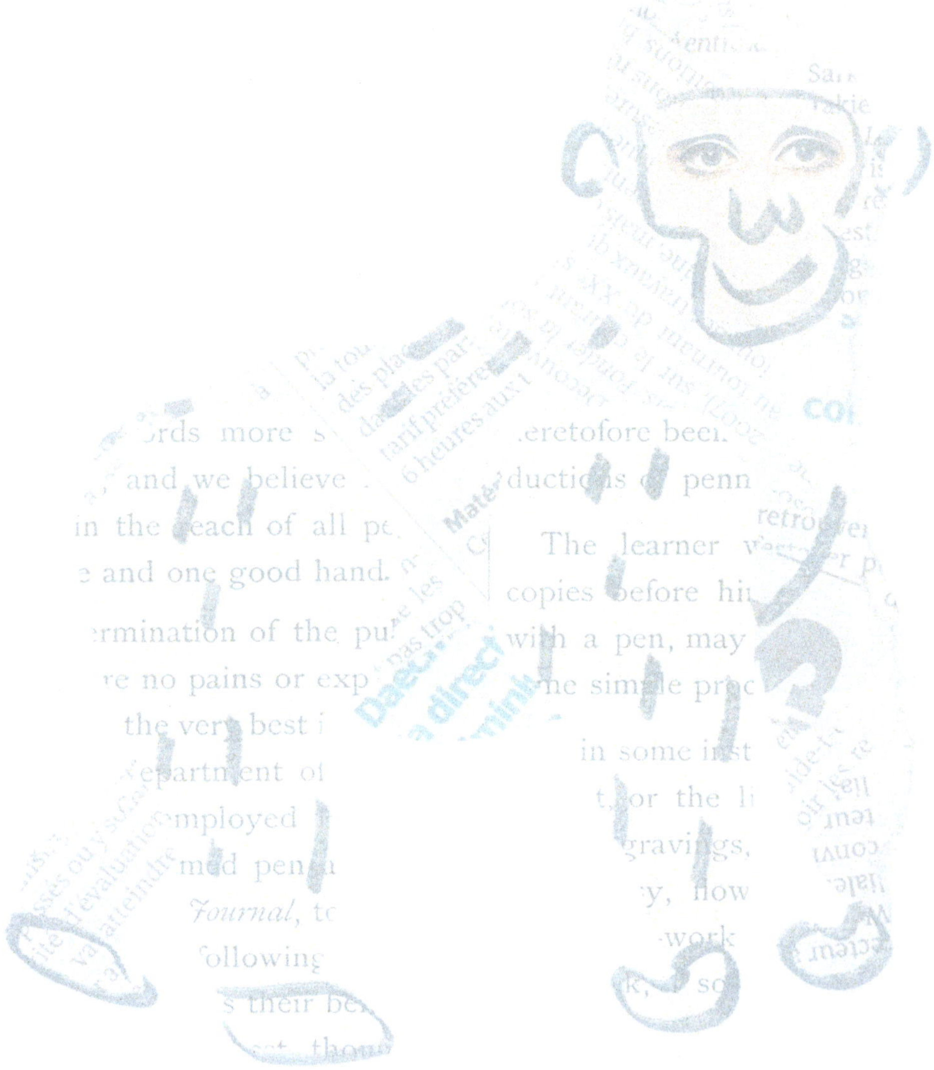

ords more s
and we believe
in the reach of all pe
e and one good hand.
rmination of the pu
re no pains or exp
the very best i
epartment of
mployed
med pen
Journal, to
following
s their be
eretofore been
ductions of penn
The learner w
copies before hi
with a pen, may
me simple proc
in some inst
t, or the l
gravings,
y, flow
-work
k, I so

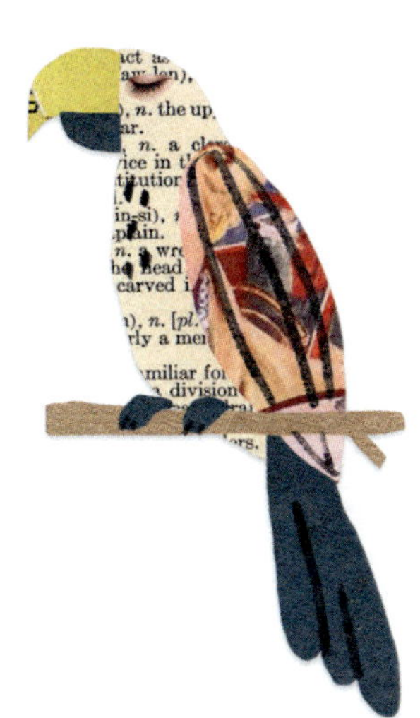

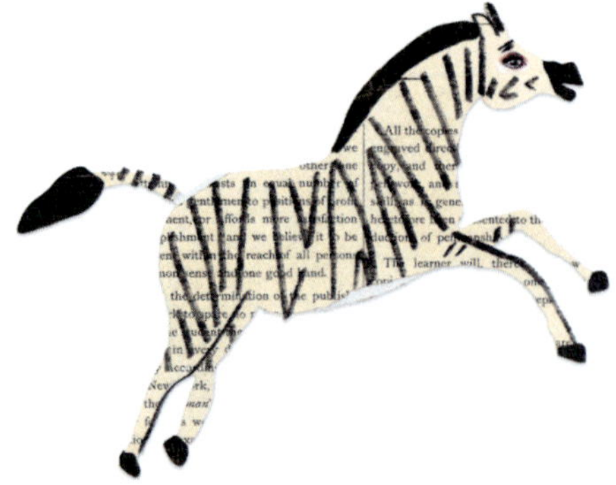

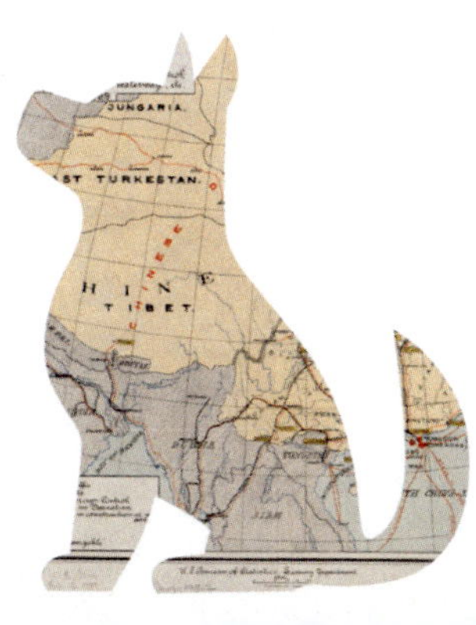
JUNGARIA
ST TURKESTAN.

This is just the beginning of your story, little one. The rest (and the best!) is yet to come.

Examples/Inspiration:

Let me tell you the beginning of your story...

You were born on:
(This section can be whatever you know about date, time, location, birth process, or other details for example:)

March 4, 2021 after 15 hours of labor.

in:
Akron, Ohio at the hospital on Main Street.

and....
My childhood doctor delivered you, you were born during a blizzard, you arrived four days early, your aunt was in the room with me when you arrived, you were the first baby born that morning.

When you were in my belly...
You kicked a lot, you got hiccups every night, I rubbed you with my hands all the time, you grew quickly, you sucked your thumb in the ultrasounds, you loved hearing music, you liked when I danced, you had your feet in my ribs, I craved mint chocolate chip ice cream, I could only eat watermelon, I was happy, I loved watching you grow, I got really big,

When I first imagined seeing you....
I felt our connection, I thought you were so beautiful, I cried, then I called my mom, I said a prayer, I couldn't believe it, I felt so many things, my heart broke a little because I would miss you, I felt nervous, I trusted the universe.

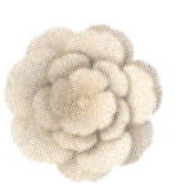

What amazed me most about you was...
You were so calm, you never stopped moving, you are beautiful, you looked right at me with your eyes, you made eye contact from the beginning, you slept peacefully, you seem so comfortable.

I want you to know that...
You are very special to me, you are worth more than you know, I will think about you all the time, we will always be connected, I will remember your birthday every year, I love you, you have a wonderful life ahead of you, I am finding you the best home I can.

Here's where I lived when I was pregnant with you....
I lived in an apartment on Martin Street, I was staying at a community center, I was living with family,

Here are some of the other places we have been...
We went to extended family's house, visited with friends, spent time at the park, I liked to go walking in my neighborhood, sometimes we just hung out at home.

This is what I know about what's next for you...
I know that you are going to a new family, I know that you'll be going into foster care, I know that you'll be adopted, I know that you'll be placed with extended family for a while, I know that you'll be going to a temporary home, I don't know.

My hopes and dreams for you are...
(This can be anything that you hope and dream for your baby from infancy, through childhood and into the future.)

I hope that you grow up feeling deeply loved and have a joyful, fulfilling life, I dream that you have all the support you need, I hope you are surrounded by friends for your whole life, My greatest wish is for you to be happy and successful and proud of who you are.

Please always remember...
You are loved, you matter, you are precious, you are the only you, I love you.

Laurie & Abby are childhood friends, sister soul mates, and now, collaborators!

Abigail Glass

Abigail Glass is a Licensed Marriage and Family Therapist, as well as a wife, mother, and healing seeker. She has personal and professional experience in the areas of fertility treatment, adoption, miscarriage and early loss, and surrogacy. Abigail's own journey helped shape her professional practice which focuses on growing and nurturing individuals and families. Her work includes supporting those who want to create a healthier emotional life, develop more fulfilling relationships, and heal from trauma, anxiety, and depression. Abigail utilizes an eclectic approach to support people in expanding their consciousness, and finding healing and hope. She is the author of *My Mom is a Surrogate*. Learn more at abigailglassmft.com.

Laurie Shiers

Laurie Shiers is a writer, an ICF Professional Certified Coach, and very proud mama bear to her amazing son who she and her husband adopted from Thailand in 2008. As a coach, Laurie helps artists and entrepreneurs break through blocks to become more self-aware, joyful, and fulfilled in all areas of their lives. She is creator of Creative Block, a tool that creatives of all kinds use to get out their own way. Laurie is also the co-author of the bestselling book, *Mindset Mondays with DTK* and is currently working on a middle grade book series about belonging.
Learn more at laurieshiers.com.

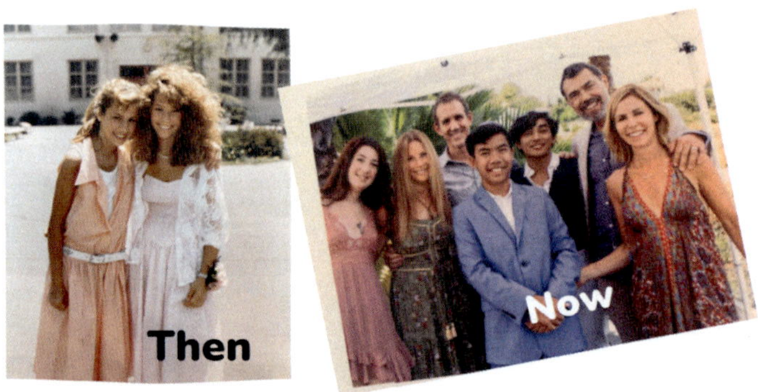

We dedicate this book series to our boys, and to YOU!

Other books by these authors

Tell Me About My Birth Father
Tell Me About My Birth Story

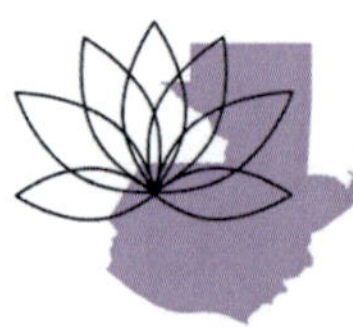

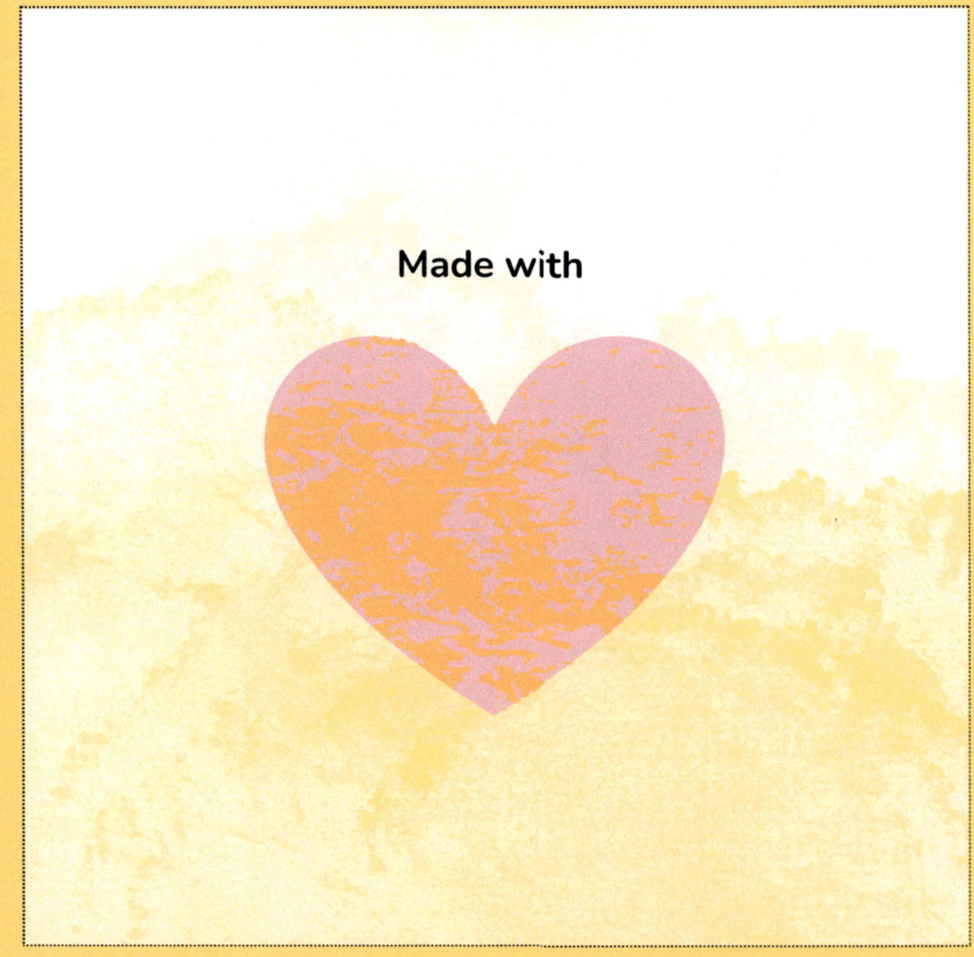
Made with

Made in the USA
Monee, IL
27 December 2024

9a23a0ae-7bae-4a8e-9c90-f7c2b667412eR01